What you really need to know about

CARING FOR A CHILD WITH ASTHMA

Dr. Robert Buckman

with Jan Hurst

Introduced by John Cleese

Macmillan Canada
Toronto

A Marshall Edition
Conceived by Marshall Editions, The Orangery, 161 New Bond Street, London W1Y 9PA

Edited and designed by Phoebus Editions, 72-80 Leather Lane, London EC1N 7TR
First published in the UK in 1999 by Marshall Publishing Ltd.

First published in Canada in 1999 by Macmillan Canada, an imprint of CDG Books Canada Inc.

Canadian Cataloguing in Publication Data
Buckman, Rob
What you really need to know about caring for a child with asthma
Includes index
ISBN 0-7715-7669-2
1. Asthma in children - Popular works. I.Cleese, John. II.Title.
III.Title: Caring for a child with asthma
RI436.A8B82 1999   618.92'238   C99-932339-3

Originated in Italy by Articolor. Printed in and bound in Italy by New Interlitho.

Project Editor Alison Murdoch, Additional Editing Jill Cropper, Indexer Stephen Fall,
Art Editor Louise Morley, Illustrator Coral Mula, Picture Research Carina Dvorak,
Managing Editor Anne Yelland, Managing Art Editor Helen Spencer, Editorial
Director Ellen Dupont, Art Director Dave Goodman, Editorial Coordinator Ros Highstead,
Production Nikki Ingram, Anna Pauletti, DTP Mike Grigoletti, Lesley Gilbert

This book is available at special discounts for bulk purchases by your group or organization for sales
promotions, premiums, fundraising and seminars. For details contact: CDG Books Canada,
99 Yorkville Avenue, Suite 400, Toronto, ON, M5R 3K5, Tel: 416-963-8830

The consultant for this book was Shari Leipzig M.D., who is an obstetrician and gynecologist in general
practice in New York City. She is also a clinical instructor of obstetrics and gynecology
at Mt. Sinai School of Medicine.

Note: In this book, we refer to your child as "he" or "she" in alternate articles. All the
information is equally applicable to both girls and boys.

1 2 3 4 5   Marshall 03 02 01 00 99

Contents

Foreword

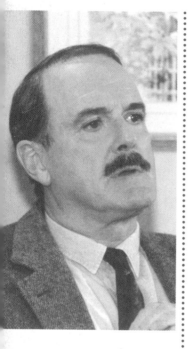

Most of you know me best as someone who makes people laugh.

But for 30 years I've also been involved with communicating information. And one particular area in which communication often breaks down is the doctor/patient relationship. We have all come across doctors who fail to communicate clearly, using complex medical terms when a simple explanation would do, and dismiss us with a "Come back in a month if you still feel unwell." Fortunately I met Dr. Robert Buckman.

Rob is one of North America's leading experts on cancer, but far more importantly he is a doctor who believes that hiding behind medical jargon is unhelpful and unprofessional. He wants his patients to understand what is wrong with them, and spends many hours with them—and their families and close friends—making sure they understand everything. Together we created a series of videos, with the jargon-free title *Videos for Patients*. Their success has prompted us to write books that explore medical conditions in the same clear, simple terms.

This book is one of a series that will tell you all you need to know, as a parent or caregiver, about your child's condition. It assumes nothing. If you have a helpful, honest, communicative doctor, you will find here the extra information that he or she simply may not have time to tell you. If you are less fortunate, this book will help to give you a much clearer picture of your situation.

More importantly—and this was a major factor in the success of the videos—you can access the information here again and again. Turn back, read over, until you really know what your doctor's diagnosis means. In addition, because in the middle of a consultation you may not think of everything you would like to ask your doctor, you can also use the book to help you formulate the questions you would like to discuss with him or her.

John Cleese

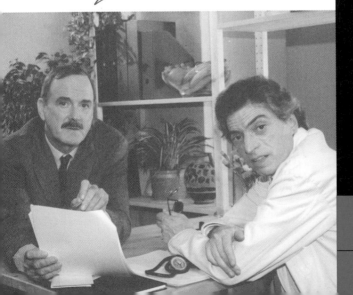

Introduction

✓ Find out as much as you can about your child's condition—with information and support you can control it together.

✗ Do not be afraid to ask questions and seek help.

Asthma is an increasingly common condition, affecting two million children in the United States. The U.S., Australia, New Zealand, and the United Kingdom have the highest rates of childhood asthma in the world.

Information and support

If you have just experienced your child's first asthma attack you may be feeling frightened and vulnerable as a parent—our first instinct is to protect our children and keep them healthy, and asthma is a threat to that. Or, if you have been living with asthma in your family for some time, you may feel that it is a burden that you cannot properly control. These feelings are very common in the parents of asthmatic children but you can and should try to overcome them.

Asthma is definitely easier to come to terms with if you have a positive attitude to it, and in order to gain that attitude you need to feel that you are in control, that you are doing all the right things, and that you know how to behave in any given situation. If you grasp control of your child's condition you will instill confidence in her and help her to accept and overcome any symptoms.

This book helps you gain control over the asthma in your family's life by answering your questions and confronting your fears; by showing you how to minimize unfavorable conditions and problems; and by explaining asthma medication and treatment and how to get the best from them.

A positive approach

Normal breathing is something most of us do without conscious effort. The result of an asthma attack is that, triggered by any of a number of causes, not enough oxygen reaches the lungs. This can result in distressing symptoms such as tightness in the chest, wheezing, or gasping for breath. In this book we will explain the various tests and indications your doctor will make use of when diagnosing your child's condition. If your doctor diagnoses asthma, it is important to remain positive— your child will look to you for guidance as to how to deal with the condition, and a practical, upbeat approach from you will rub off on her.

A normal life

An asthmatic child needs to find out, with your help and support, how to control her condition so that she can enjoy a happy, active childhood. There is no reason why she cannot join in any school activities that interest her and she need not feel "different" from her friends.

The goal is to establish a balance between prevention and relief medication so that your child experiences the absolute minimum of symptoms for her degree of asthma. With the right kind of practical care and a positive approach, there is every chance that she will grow up as healthy and active as any other child.

SELF-HELP PROGRAMS

There are many programs throughout the United States and Canada to help children and families become more self-sufficient in their handling of the asthma in their lives. See addresses on page 78.

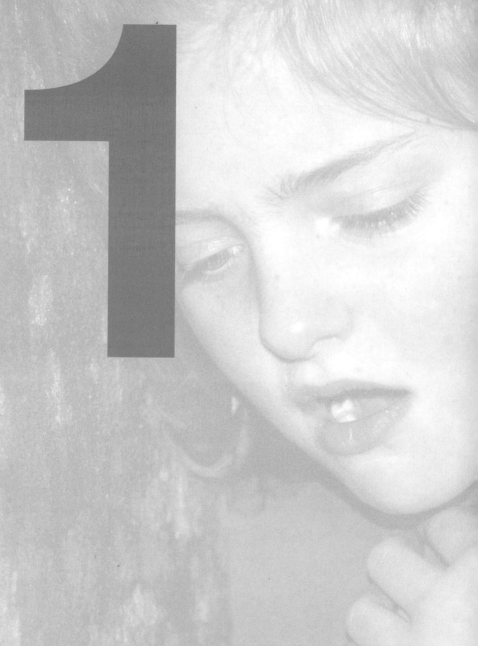

Chapter

1

SYMPTOMS & CAUSES

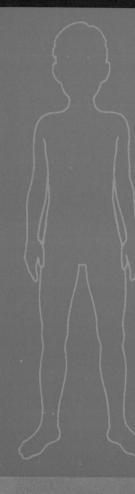

What is asthma?

Asthma is a condition in which the small airways in the lungs (the bronchioles) narrow to such a point that normal breathing becomes difficult.

This constriction or narrowing stops when treatment is given and the airways go back to their normal size when the asthma attack is over. It is the sound of the air squeezing through the narrowed tubes that makes the wheezing sound commonly associated with asthma.

What makes the airways narrow?

Three main actions cause the airways to narrow and allow less air to pass through. In the first, the walls of the airways, which are made from muscle, contract and restrict the available space for the air to flow through.

HOW AIR ENTERS AND LEAVES THE LUNGS

The lungs fill most of the space in the chest. Air is drawn into the lungs when the muscular diaphragm below them contracts. The air travels down the windpipe (trachea), into the large and small airways (the bronchi and bronchioles) and then into the air sacs (alveoli), where oxygen is delivered into and carbon dioxide is taken from the blood. The diaphragm then relaxes and the carbon dioxide travels back through the lungs and is exhaled.

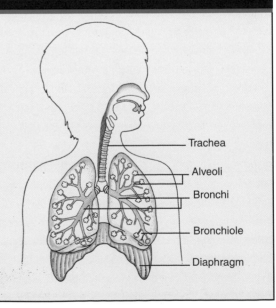

Trachea

Alveoli

Bronchi

Bronchiole

Diaphragm

Secondly, the lining of the airways becomes inflamed, further reducing the space within the airways.

Thirdly, the mucus secretions that are always present in the lungs increase in volume during some attacks, and the sufferer cannot cough them away. If a child is suffering from a cold or other respiratory infection, this can often trigger an attack.

Why are children so affected?

Children's lungs are smaller and the airways are narrower than those of an adult, making the effects of the three actions more pronounced. This partly explains why many asthmatic children are completely free of the condition by the time they reach adulthood.

What causes an asthma attack?

In the normal course of events, asthma is a chronic (ongoing) though "invisible" condition: An asthmatic child will be equally able to enjoy life and take part in activities alongside her non-asthmatic friends, until something "triggers" her asthma symptoms.

There are many asthma triggers. Some individuals are affected by just a few; others by a wide range. The most common include those that are inhaled during normal breathing, such as pollen, dust, pollution, perfumes, extremely cold air, and cigarette smoke. In some cases, certain foods can provoke an allergic reaction. Attacks can be caused by emotions: Some asthmatics react to stress or fears in themselves or those close to them, and some will even suffer an onset of wheezing from a prolonged bout of laughter. In some cases, an attack follows an infection and inflammation of the lungs. Exercise is another common trigger.

YOU REALLY NEED TO KNOW

◆ In many children asthma attacks are less frequent as they grow older; some outgrow the condition completely.

◆ Most asthma symptoms can be safely and successfully dealt with at home.

◆ The more you understand about asthma and how to treat it, the easier it will become to stop attacks occurring in the first place.

What is asthma?

What happens in an attack?

SELF-HELP

Learning to identify the early signs of an attack allows you to treat it before it becomes more serious.

Wheezing does not necessarily mean that an attack is at an advanced stage.

What actually happens in an asthma attack varies quite a lot according to each individual and the severity and frequency of the attacks they normally suffer, but the common feature is an inability to breathe normally.

How does an attack begin?

An attack may begin gradually or abruptly. The first signs are often shortness of breath and the child may breathe faster and with more effort in an attempt to get more air into his lungs. He may also wheeze and cough, show signs of anxiety, and pant as he talks. Breathing out is more difficult than breathing in, so he may hunch forward to make breathing easier and you will probably hear the characteristic wheezing noise as he breathes out.

HOW TO HELP YOUR CHILD DURING AN ATTACK

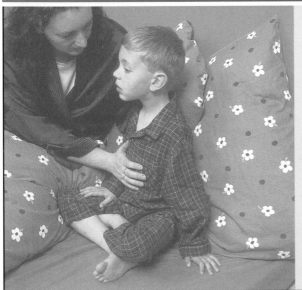

Being unable to get his breath can be a very frightening experience for a child. Although you may also feel alarmed, it is vital to stay calm so that he does not react to your feelings and panic and start to hyperventilate. If the attack happens when the child is in bed, help him to sit upright, perhaps propped up with pillows, to make it easier for air to reach the lungs.

With children, especially very young children, the onset of an asthma attack can sometimes be difficult to recognize. But if you can learn to identify the early stages of an attack in your child you will be able to deal with it before it worsens and, usually, prevent it from developing into a more serious attack.

What causes a child's first attack?

A first attack may come on without obvious cause, or it may be preceded by a cold or chest infection that has led to excess mucus accumulating in the airways. If the attack is severe you may need to call your child's doctor or even go immediately to the nearest hospital emergency room. Even if it is less severe you should still contact your doctor as soon as possible because your child needs to be examined medically to make sure there are no other problems that require treatment.

What are the early warning signs?

If your child has already been diagnosed as asthmatic you may notice that an attack nearly always begins in the same way. Many parents say that coughing during the night is the first sign of an impending asthma attack—the cough will not be relieved by a drink of water, although it may be eased temporarily by propping the child up in bed with more pillows.

Will my child wheeze?

Wheezing indicates that the air is not flowing easily through your child's airways so it is quite usual for him to wheeze at the beginning of an attack. It may sound alarming, but wheezing does not necessarily mean that the attack is already at a serious stage.

YOU REALLY NEED TO KNOW

◆ Indicators that an attack is taking place include faster breathing, increased coughing (particularly at night), and wheezing. Breathing also takes more effort.

◆ Even if you deal with an asthma attack easily and it passes quickly you should still make an appointment with your child's doctor.

◆ Children who have severe attacks and are hospitalized when very young can still "grow out" of the condition completely.

What happens in an attack?

Why should I breastfeed?

BREASTFEEDING

✓ If you are finding breastfeeding difficult, ask at your doctor's office for the contact number of a local breastfeeding counselor or local lactation support group.

✓ Breastfeeding works by supply and demand. The more you feed your baby, the more milk you will make.

Research indicates that babies who are breastfed are less likely to develop eczema or other allergy-related conditions. If you, your partner, an older child or other close family members suffer from asthma or other allergy-related problems there is a higher than average chance that your child will also do so. It is, therefore, well worth breastfeeding your baby if you can and continuing to do so for as long as possible.

How can breastfeeding help?

Experts are still not sure exactly how breast milk acts as a protection against asthma, but it is known that breast milk contains high levels of antibodies. These antibodies provide the walls of the baby's intestines with a protective lining in the first few days after birth. Formula milk mimics breast milk in many ways but it cannot reproduce these natural antibodies.

How long should I breastfeed?

It is advisable, when you have a family history of atopy (see p. 20), to breastfeed for six months and to keep your baby's diet to breast milk alone during that time. There is often pressure from other new parents and from older members of the family to introduce "solids," in the hope your baby will sleep through the night, or because they are concerned that she may not be getting enough nourishment. But there is no evidence to suggest early weaning solves sleep, or indeed any other, problems.

If your baby is hungry she will naturally be able to stimulate a greater supply of breast milk to satisfy her requirements—all you need to do is to eat a healthy, satisfying amount of food, get plenty of rest, and feed your baby as often as she demands it.

Will weaning be difficult?

When you know that your baby has an increased risk of asthma, you can plan ahead and take some sensible precautions when you begin introducing your baby to solid foods. Fortunately, this does not mean you have to search out difficult to find, expensive food items or spend a long time cooking special meals for your baby. It simply means following a few basic rules.

SUCCESSFUL WEANING

Start by feeding your child baby rice, but mix it with some puréed fruit, such as banana, apple, or pear, or with expressed breast milk or baby formula milk. Offer yogurt and cheese once your baby is used to having a variety of foods, from about six months. Well-cooked egg yolk can be introduced from eight months, but if possible delay introducing egg white until your child is a year old. Avoid giving cow's milk until your baby is at least one year old.

Do not introduce wheat until your child is at least seven months old. This means initially avoiding many foods, such as breads and cereals; choose from the wide variety of gluten-free products that are available instead.

Introduce all new foods to your baby slowly and separately, ideally at least a week apart. Apart from giving your baby time to get used to new tastes, this makes it easier to identify the culprit if an allergic reaction does occur.

YOU REALLY NEED TO KNOW

◆ Experts strongly recommend breastfeeding for at least the first twelve weeks, longer if possible.

◆ Signs that your baby may be allergic to certain foods may include skin rash, puffiness around the eyes or mouth, a red bottom, vomiting, and diarrhea.

◆ Avoid giving your child all nuts and peanuts for at least two years. If there is a strong family history of allergies or eczema, it is better to avoid them for the first five years.

Why should I breastfeed?

Points to remember

There are six vitally important points to share with your child: how to take control of the condition, prevent attacks, seek help at school and elsewhere, use medication correctly, recognize when medical help is needed and take responsibility. They are the key to your asthmatic child enjoying good health.

✓ The amount of control your child will be able to take depends on his age and on his attitude to his condition.

✓ Learn to go with your gut reaction to make a quick assessment of your child's condition.

✗ Don't nag or be over-protective since this will probably only make your child rebel.

1. Help your child to take control

Only by knowing how to control his condition will your child be able to stop it controlling him. You have to be confident about how the medication he has been prescribed works, and how it needs to be taken to be most effective, so that you can pass this information on.

Control is achieved through the right medication in the correct amounts, taken at the right time, using an appropriate age-related device. A healthy diet and

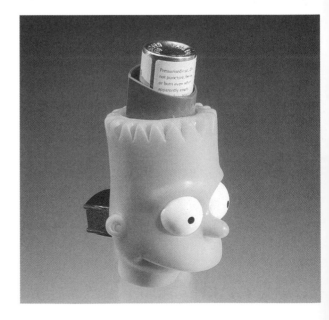

A humorous inhaler cover, such as this "Bart Simpson" design, may make your child feel less self-conscious about using his medication in public or in front of his friends. Many larger pharmacies stock a range of covers.

lifestyle, while not directly affecting your child's asthma, will ensure that he is fit and can fight infection.

Talk to your child to discover when he feels vulnerable because of asthma. You can then work with him to find ways that situations can be improved, and how to help him to remember to take his medication at the correct times. It is also important that he knows to stop physical play and exercise when and if he needs to.

2. Concentrate on prevention

As you help your child to understand his asthma you will also be showing him how to prevent attacks. A good time to talk to him is when he is relatively asthma-free. Try to get him to acknowledge what triggers an attack and what to do about it. Suggest that he works out an asthma plan—your asthma nurse or doctor could help. Make it clear that he is in control and you have complete confidence in him, but that he can talk to you at any time about anything that worries him.

Your child may be unwilling for you to include his school in any plan of prevention. While you can sympathize with his dread of being singled out, be honest and say that you have to inform the school of his condition and explain how they can help.

3. Know when to tell someone

Teaching your child to tell somebody if he feels he is losing control over his asthma can be quite difficult. You must help him overcome any worries he may have about communicating his needs to an adult. Pave the way by making sure staff at his school are informed, and that parents of friends he visits understand. It is vital your child learns to tell somebody, sooner rather than later.

YOU REALLY NEED TO KNOW

◆ Don't always wait for your child to begin wheezing before you give medication. If you know a cold could trigger an attack, or if he has been in contact with another trigger, medicate him whether or not symptoms are apparent.

◆ Teach your child to "be calm, be polite, but be firm." If he is in any doubt that the adult he has told has not taken him seriously, he should seek help from someone else.

◆ Contact an asthma society or support group for information you can give to the staff at your child's school.

Points to remember

Points to remember

Make sure your child's school has an up-to-date contact number for you and for your child's doctor.

Your child should also memorize your telephone number and details of his medication.

4. Use medication correctly

Medication only works if taken at the right times and in the right amounts. If your child has had an attack after taking medication he may have lost faith in it. Help him by cultivating a routine in which he takes his maintenance medication, if prescribed, just before he brushes his teeth.

Inhalers that alleviate asthmatic symptoms also need to be used properly. Your child should know why they are important and he needs to understand that he should turn to them as his first, rather than a last, resort. It is also important not to overuse or abuse relievers and to watch his response carefully. If his response is poor or lasts for less than four hours, seek medical help without delay.

HELP YOUR CHILD MAKE AN ASTHMA PLAN

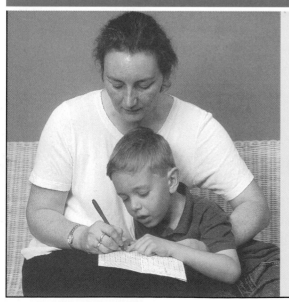

No matter how attentive you are, you won't be with your child every time he has an asthma attack. This makes it doubly important that your child learns to cope with his condition and feels confident about all aspects of the management of his asthma. Making an asthma plan is a crucial part of this education, and doing so will reassure him and make him feel more in control of his condition.

5. Know when to get medical help

However efficiently you both manage to control your child's asthma there will probably still be times when he needs medical attention. While it is important not to show fear to your child, who may become worse if you do, or to overreact to his symptoms, it is essential to heed warning signs and to act promptly.

If your child has been hospitalized before, he may try to avoid it happening again, and so conceal the seriousness of the attack, but you must be objective. If his usual medication has not given any significant relief at the start of the attack, it is not likely to do so later. It is vital that your child's medication should be accessible at all times, but if he does come into contact with triggers that have caused an attack before and does not have his medication with him, contact your doctor right away.

Plan ahead. If you receive a telephone call from your child's school to say he is ill from asthma, telephone your doctor's office before you leave to pick him up. Don't be afraid to insist that your child needs immediate attention—a child having an asthma attack is a priority.

6. Pass on information

As your child grows up, he will gradually become more independent and start to take more responsibility for his condition. The more he knows and the more confident he feels, the easier this will be.

It is more difficult for a child to make himself heard than it is for an adult, but he will stand a much better chance if it is apparent that he understands his asthma and knows what needs to be done. But be careful not to alarm your child: Your aim is to educate him about his asthma without making him afraid of his condition.

YOU REALLY NEED TO KNOW

◆ Keep your doctor's telephone number with you at all times and know the fastest route to the hospital. Always have enough gas in the tank. If you are prepared for emergencies, you are more likely to stay calm.

◆ Make sure your child's asthma plan is up to date. Regularly talk to the asthma nurse or your doctor and revise your routine, if necessary.

◆ Get to know the parents of other asthmatics; your child will be reassured to know how common the condition is.

Points to remember

What is atopy?

✓ Cotton clothing is best for sensitive skin. Wash fabrics with laundry detergents formulated for sensitive skins and rinse them thoroughly.

✗ Don't use soap on the skin of children suffering from eczema or dermatitis. Special emulsifying creams can be used instead.

Atopy means having an inherited likelihood of developing the conditions of asthma, eczema, infantile dermatitis, hay fever, and allergic rhinitis. Many children with asthma also have one or more of the other atopic conditions and the presence of one indicates a higher likelihood of developing one or more of the others.

Eczema

Atopic eczema usually develops from around two months old. It appears as red patches on the cheeks, arms and legs, or body. Eczema is very irritating and it can be difficult to prevent the scratching which can lead to infection.

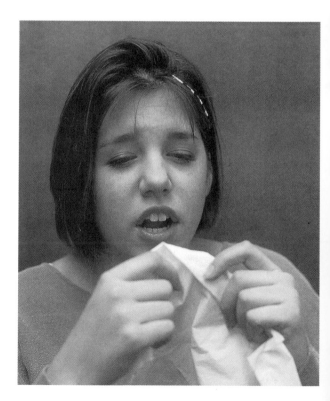

Most hay fever attacks are provoked by grass pollen, which is most abundant from late spring to late summer. Some sufferers also react to tree pollen, which is released in spring, and to weed pollen, which is common in spring and fall.

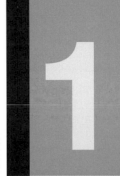

Although atopic eczema is inherited, it can be made worse by allergic reactions following skin contact with such things as wool, laundry detergents, and soaps. For persistent eczema, a mild steroid cream can be prescribed, and if an infection has set in, antibiotics as well. Eczema frequently disappears as children get older.

Dermatitis

This atopic condition can appear in babies as diaper rash or as seborrheic dermatitis. Seborrheic dermatitis looks red and weepy and affects the forehead, nose, eyelids, scalp, and behind the ears. It appears in the first few weeks of life and can indicate that eczema will develop. Dermatitis is aggravated by soap and rough fabrics.

Hay fever

Children are not usually affected by hay fever (a pollen allergy) until they are between five and ten years old. If your child has atopic asthma she may also have a runny nose; profuse sneezing; swollen, itchy eyelids; and a cough during summer—this is hay fever. Although relatively harmless in itself, hay fever can provoke an asthma attack, so you need to be vigilant.

Allergic rhinitis

Hay fever is seasonal but allergic rhinitis can happen throughout the year, whenever the mucous membrane lining inside the nose is affected by other allergy-causing substances, such as dust, feathers, fur, smoke, or fungi spores. The symptoms include a blocked, runny nose, which can be treated with a nasal spray containing locally acting steroids. They may also be helped by taking an anti-histamine by mouth.

YOU REALLY NEED TO KNOW

◆ Several different sprays and drops are available for hay fever and allergic rhinitis. If your child finds one stings too much, ask for a different type.

◆ It is very unlikely your child will suffer from all the atopic conditions described, and certainly not all at once.

◆ Atopic eczema should be taken as an early warning that asthma may be on the horizon, otherwise the first asthma attack may be misread as bronchitis or a chest infection.

What is atopy?

All about atopy

✓ Once you have decided which practical steps to take to minimize your child's risk of developing allergies, try to stop worrying about the subject.

✓ If you do not fully understand everything your doctor has told you, go back and ask again until you do. Find out if written information is available.

✓ Do your best to treat your children equally, and try not to be overprotective toward the one with atopic allergies.

If your doctor tells you your child is atopic, you may feel worried. Does this mean that his asthma is inherited and that there's nothing you can do about it? Or worse still, that he will be allergic to everything?

Happily, the answer to both of these questions is "No." Atopy simply means that an individual has a genetic predisposition to developing allergies and asthma because these run in the family. Not all children develop symptoms, however, and even if they do, there is much that can be done to help.

How are allergies inherited?

Atopy is a genetically inherited syndrome due to not one but several genes that determine whether or not a child will inherit a condition, and whether the condition, once inherited, will be serious or mild.

For example, if you have non-identical twins, only one may develop atopic asthma, while the other may just have mild eczema, or even nothing at all.

This explains why atopic asthma may seem almost random in a family. In many cases, though, even if only one child is seriously affected by asthma, other children in the family will probably have had bouts of eczema, hay fever, or dermatitis.

Can asthma be predicted?

About 10-15 percent of all babies develop asthma and the likelihood is higher in families with a history of atopy. If one parent is atopic, the likelihood of his or her baby developing asthma is about 30 percent. If both parents are atopic, the tendency increases to about 50 percent. In addition, if a baby suffers from eczema, there is a strong chance that he will go on to develop asthma.

Is there anything I can do?

While there is nothing you can do to be absolutely sure that asthma will not manifest itself in your child, there are a number of sensible, easy precautions that you can take to make it either less likely to develop or, if it does appear, to keep symptoms to a minimum. These precautions, which you will find on the following pages, involve planning ahead and making a number of relatively simple changes to your home and lifestyle.

IDENTICAL TWINS AND ATOPY

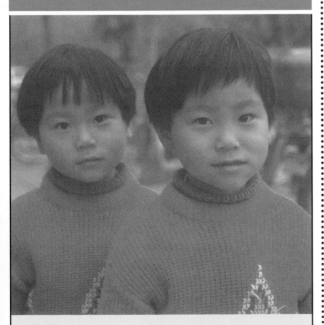

Identical twins are always either both atopic or both non-atopic. Even if both are atopic, however, one may go on to develop allergies while the other remains unaffected.

1

YOU REALLY NEED TO KNOW

◆ You should not be alarmed by family scare stories regarding atopic asthma—treatments have vastly improved in recent years, and if you are forewarned you are forearmed.

◆ If you are not sure that you have discovered all the triggers for your child's condition, do a little detective work among family members who also have asthma.

◆ Until puberty, boys are twice as likely to be affected by asthma than girls. The incidence then becomes similar in both sexes.

All about atopy

Common asthma triggers

Get into the habit of consulting the advance weather forecasts so that you can plan your child's activities and keep her indoors if necessary.

Moving your child's bedroom from the front to the back of the house may reduce the level of exhaust fumes reaching her and hence affect the frequency and severity of her attacks.

You may feel that the substances or conditions that make an asthma attack more likely, or those that trigger a full-blown attack in your child, form an ever-growing and difficult-to-handle list. On the plus side, however, the more you know about possible triggers the easier it is to use avoidance tactics to protect your child.

Outdoor irritants

If you live in an urban area, two possible triggers your child will come into contact with are traffic pollution and, at certain times of year and with certain weather conditions, low-level ozone. You can help your child by staying away from traffic-congested streets as much as possible. It is also worth checking the reports of ozone levels given out in the press and on the radio and TV, so that you can keep her indoors when air quality is poor.

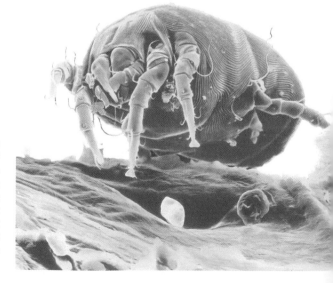

Dust mites are minute eight-legged relatives of spiders that feed on the dead scales of human skin in household dust. Millions exist in even the cleanest home and are the most common—and most difficult to eradicate—asthma trigger.

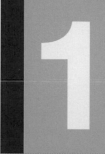

If your house is on a very busy main road you should make sure your child's bedroom faces away from the road and ever-present exhaust fumes. You may consider moving, but the countryside may not necessarily be the answer: fields of pollen-laden crops, intensive farming, and the chemicals that are now in widespread use can also act as asthma triggers.

If your child suffers from hay fever, it's worth remembering, when planning a picnic in the country, to choose your site carefully so you do not end up sitting close to a field of hay or on freshly cut grass.

Weather conditions

Extremes of temperature can affect asthmatics in a number of ways. Moving from warm to cold conditions and vice versa can irritate oversensitive airways, so if you take your child skiing, or even just outside on a cold day, make sure she has her inhaler handy. Similarly, avoid stepping out of a cool, air-conditioned room into a hot, dusty street whenever possible.

It is also useful to know that certain weather combinations can have an adverse effect on many asthma sufferers. Hot and humid summer days, when a storm is threatening, especially in city conditions, almost always signify an unusually high number of patients being treated for asthma attacks in hospital emergency rooms.

House dust

The most common inhaled trigger is house dust, specifically the part of it that contains the feces of the tiny house dust mites that are found in every home, no matter how often and how thoroughly it is cleaned.

Common asthma triggers

✓ Teach your child not to linger in smoky atmospheres and never to start smoking herself.

✓ Help your child to recognize the point at which a giggling fit is getting out of control so she can calm herself down.

✗ If you think your child may be suffering from a food allergy, write down everything she eats for a couple of weeks, and her symptoms. But don't eliminate foods from her diet before consulting an expert.

Pets, smoke, and mold

Second only to dust mites as a trigger is pet dander—the fur, hair, and accumulated dust that is shed mainly by cats and dogs but also by other pets, such as guinea pigs, hamsters, and rabbits.

Cigarette smoke is another serious inhaled trigger. Passive smoking (breathing in other people's smoke) is particularly harmful to asthmatic children because it gives their respiratory systems an extra burden to cope with.

The mold and spores that thrive in damp conditions can also trigger an attack in susceptible individuals.

Food allergies

If your child has an allergy to a particular food and is asthmatic, part of her allergic reaction may involve asthmatic symptoms. An allergic reaction can be quite dramatic with, for example, a red blotchy rash, vomiting, and puffy face. It always happens immediately so you will almost certainly be able to pinpoint the cause.

Food allergies are associated with all the atopic conditions already mentioned (see p. 20), though they are a much less common trigger than inhaled irritants. It is best to be guided by your instincts and to seek medical help if you feel it is necessary.

Other illnesses

If your child has a viral infection, such as a cold or bronchitis, you may find that a bout of asthma follows close on its heels. This is because the airways, which are already affected by her asthma, are now under attack from the infection as well. Colds in very young children quite often lead to an asthma attack, sometimes through a build-up of mucus in the airways.

THE EFFECTS OF EMOTIONS

Just as many physical factors can trigger an asthma attack, so can extremes of feeling, such as stress, overexcitement, and sadness.

It is now recognized that even young children react to stressful situations, such as parental splits and exam pressures at school, in the same way that adults do. Real stress makes physical demands on the body—blood pressure rises, muscles tense, and the breathing rate speeds up.

In the same way, feelings of excitement or fear, or even a long bout of hysterical laughter, all of which make an increased demand on the child's lungs, can make an asthma attack more likely.

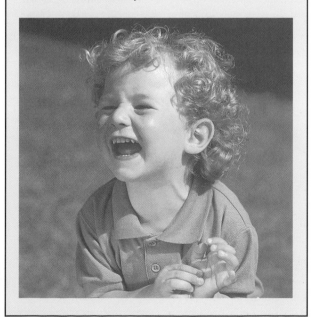

YOU REALLY NEED TO KNOW

◆ Research indicates that frequent house moves contribute to childhood asthma. This could be due to being exposed to an ever-changing range of triggers.

◆ Mold spores are found both indoors and outdoors. They are equally prevalent in the spring, summer and fall, so it can be difficult to establish whether an individual is reacting to mold or pollen.

Common asthma triggers

Common asthma triggers

✓ Ask your doctor for advice if you are concerned that your child might be overweight.

✓ Encourage an overweight child to get more exercise and to avoid eating "empty calories," such as sweets and sodas.

✗ Never put your child on a reduced calorie diet without getting medical advice.

Reducing the risks

There is always the temptation to try to protect an asthmatic child from anything that might provoke an attack, but your child will not benefit from overprotection and could easily end up losing confidence in her ability to be like other children.

It is difficult to avoid colds without seriously restricting your asthmatic child's freedom, especially if

EXERCISE AND ASTHMA ATTACKS

It is not uncommon for children to have an asthma attack that is brought on by exercise. This naturally causes a dilemma for parents who would not wish to provoke unnecessary attacks yet who want their child to be fit and to gain satisfaction and fun from getting exercise. As a parent you will know how enthusiastic children generally are about taking part in organized sports and playing in the park, backyard, or street with their friends.

WHO IS AFFECTED?

If your child is asthmatic she has about an 80 percent chance of her condition being affected by the physical demands of exercise. Nevertheless, exercise is definitely not out of the question. You will be able to tell her that quite a number of Olympic-standard athletes and professional sportspeople are asthmatics who have learned to control their condition. Many asthmatic people find that if they use an inhaler fifteen minutes before starting to exercise, they can prevent an attack altogether.

you have other children who will bring germs home from school. However, you can avoid visiting friends and family when they have heavy colds.

Your child's asthma should not be affected by other common childhood ailments, such as chicken pox, so you do not need to go out of your way to avoid them.

Being overweight can make asthma symptoms worse and this is worth keeping an eye on.

Generally speaking, the benefits to be gained from regular exercise outweigh the risks for asthmatics. This is principally because the more in shape and stronger your child becomes as she grows, the less likely she is to succumb to asthma symptoms.

PLANNING AHEAD

At school your child will know when she will be getting exercise and should be able to time her use of presport medication so that it is most effective. If, for some reason, she forgets and experiences tightness in the chest and wheezing she should stop exercising immediately, take her medication, and rest quietly until all her symptoms have disappeared before she starts to exercise again.

If your child finds that one form of exercise, for example running, baseball, or field hockey, always brings on an asthma attack, encourage her to take up another activity, such as swimming or yoga, which helps with breathing control.

YOU REALLY NEED TO KNOW

◆ Exposure to tobacco smoke increases the risk of developing respiratory problems, such as asthma, by about 50 percent.

◆ Yoga is an effective way of relieving stress and aiding breathing techniques.

◆ You should never replace your child's medication with an "alternative" unless you have consulted your doctor first.

◆ Try not to discuss your child's asthma with your partner or any other adults within her hearing and don't talk about her in her presence. This may make her feel frustrated by her condition.

Common asthma triggers

Chapter

2

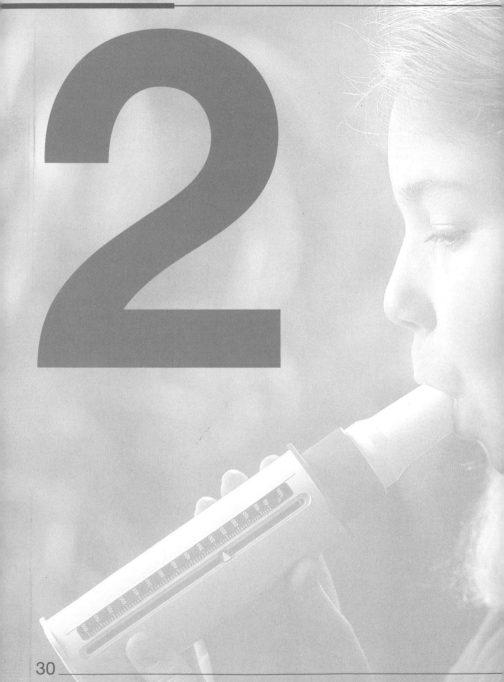

DIAGNOSIS & ASSESSMENT

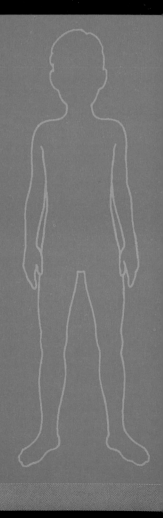

Confirming the diagnosis

✔ A persistent cough at night or after exercise is one of the most common indicators of asthma.

✔ A family history of atopic conditions, such as hay fever or eczema, should alert you to the possibility of asthma in your child.

✗ Never ignore your child's persistent cough or wheezing in the hope that it will go away on its own.

Because you know your child so well, you are most likely to spot any symptoms of asthma. You should try to remember the symptoms in detail since by the time the doctor sees your child they will probably have passed.

Diagnosing asthma

A cough, particularly a persistent cough that occurs during the night or after exercise, is one of the most common indicators. Wheezing is another sign, and suggests that the airways may be constricted. Shortness of breath, when your child has to stop what she is doing or sit up in bed in order to breathe more easily, should also be reported to your doctor, as should complaints about tight feelings in the chest.

If every cold your child catches becomes a more serious infection for which antibiotics have to be given, this could be significant to the diagnosis, especially if the antibiotics do not alleviate the condition.

Supporting evidence

Your doctor will also be looking for other information that would support a diagnosis of asthma. Tell him or her if your child has suffered from eczema or dermatitis, even if she was treated for it and it is on her medical records. You may also be asked about your family's medical history: Whether you or your partner, or your child's grandparents, have any atopic conditions, such as asthma, hay fever, dermatitis, or eczema.

Making an assessment

Once asthma has been diagnosed your doctor will want to make an assessment of its severity. Asthma varies enormously from rare bouts of wheezing to severe

KEEP A WRITTEN RECORD

Once you realize that asthma is a possibility, it will help your doctor to make an accurate diagnosis if you keep a written record of when your child felt wheezy or was coughing, or short of breath. If you keep a detailed record of her symptoms over a period of time, you and the doctor will be able to build up a pattern in order to establish what triggers the attacks.

Note exactly what her symptoms were, what time they occurred, how severe they were, and how long they lasted. It is also worth jotting down what your child was doing when the symptoms occurred—perhaps after running outside or while asleep at night—and what she had been eating. At this stage, make your notes too extensive rather than too brief; your doctor will appreciate as much information about your child as possible.

symptoms requiring repeated hospital stays. If your child is more than five years old your doctor may take a "peak flow reading" (see more on p. 34).

A peak flow meter measures how fast air leaves the lungs when your child breathes out. The doctor will probably ask her to do it two or three times to get the best reading, against which all future readings will be compared. Once he has a baseline reading he will ask you to monitor your child's peak flow at home and keep a record of it so that he can compare it after your child has been taking asthma medication. If your child's peak flow improves when she receives medication and her symptoms disappear, a diagnosis of asthma is likely.

YOU REALLY NEED TO KNOW

Some illnesses can be mistaken for asthma, especially in very young children. These include:

◆ Whooping cough—less common nowadays due to vaccination. Symptoms are severe coughing, vomiting, breathlessness, nose bleeds, and a high temperature.

◆ Cystic fibrosis—a genetic condition in which the lungs produce too much sticky mucus, which leads to recurrent chest infections.

◆ Croup—infection which comes from a cold and affects the larynx (voice box). A barking cough and breathlessness follow.

Confirming the diagnosis

Peak flow meters

The peak flow meter is a simple but very useful tool to help you manage your child's asthma. It enables you to assess her condition objectively at any given time.

What is a peak flow meter?

A peak flow meter consists of a plastic tube with a long, thin slit, against which there is a line of measurements in liters per minute. A pointer inside the meter is moved by blowing into the mouthpiece, and the distance it moves gauges the force of your child's exhalation (out breath). The mouthpiece can be removed for washing.

Your doctor will explain how readings should be done, and provide a chart to record them. Peak flow meters come in two sizes: a larger adult version (0-800l/min) and a smaller child-sized version (0-400l/min).

How do I take a reading?

You will probably be asked to take a reading in the morning after breakfast and before bedtime, every day. Your child should be standing upright. She may prefer to hold the meter herself, but you need to make absolutely sure her fingers aren't touching the gauge. Teach her to breathe in as deeply as possible, then to blow a sharp, rapid breath into the meter. Note the reading then ask her to do it again. Write the highest reading on your chart. Remember, and remind your child, that there can be a variation of around 15 percent or more between two readings and that dips often occur early in the morning. You should stress that fictitious or made-up readings are of no help to anyone.

Don't try to take peak flow readings from a child under the age of five because she will be too young to manage the routine.

What does the reading mean?

Your doctor will tell you the peak flow reading to expect when your child is healthy. You can also ask what number or range on the gauge indicates that your child's symptoms are becoming serious. Write the numbers down next to your doctor's telephone number.

The aim is to get consistent normal readings over a long period of time. If you are getting fluctuating readings over two days or more this could be an indication of an asthma attack, so watch out for other symptoms and contact your doctor for advice. Once you have established a routine with the peak flow meter you will find it very helpful in monitoring your child's condition.

A MEASURE OF BREATHING

A peak flow meter is used to monitor the efficiency of your child's lungs and can give early warning of an asthma attack. Measurement often becomes part of your morning and evening routine but once the asthma seems stable, it may be reserved for monitoring during an asthma attack.

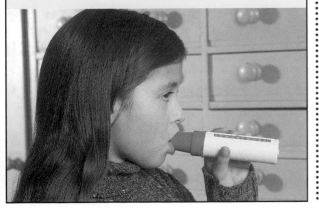

YOU REALLY NEED TO KNOW

◆ If your child is being given emergency treatment it will help the doctors to know how the attack has built up, so remember to take her peak flow chart with you.

◆ If your child's condition is worsening it is useful to take a peak flow reading, but do not repeat this too often because it can cause panic and discomfort.

◆ You can get replacement mouthpieces for the peak flow meter if yours becomes chewed or damaged.

◆ Supply your child's school with a peak flow meter like the one you normally use, on which normal and danger levels are clearly indicated.

Peak flow meters

Lung, skin, and blood tests

SELF-HELP

✓ If you suspect one particular substance is a trigger for attacks, mention this to your doctor so it can be tested first.

✓ If you don't understand what a test is or why it is being done, ask the medical staff for more information.

The most basic and useful test to measure your child's lung function is the peak flow test (see pp. 32–35), which you can carry out at home. If your child's asthma becomes more serious and he has repeated attacks, your doctor may wish to carry out further tests; these are, however, rarely necessary for most asthmatic children.

Lung function tests

Your child may be referred to an asthma or allergy specialist, who may want to see more detailed lung function readings and will carry out a pulmonary function test (PFT) using a spirometer. A spirometer is a more sophisticated version of a peak flow meter and the test is no more likely to upset your child than the peak flow test.

HOW A SKIN TEST WORKS

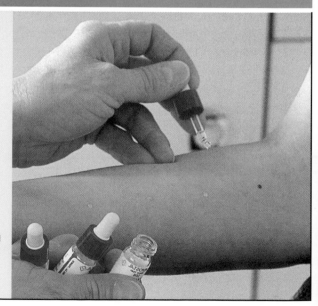

In skin-prick testing, the nurse applies drops of various common allergens, such as pollen, dust, and fungal spores, along different points on the child's arm. She then makes a small prick through the substance into the skin. Any skin inflammation indicates an immune response, showing that the patient may be allergic to that substance.

Skin tests

If your child's asthma is obviously atopic and it is proving difficult to identify what is triggering it, he may be given skin-prick tests. Tiny quantities of substances known to trigger asthma are placed on his skin and a small prick is made through the substance into the skin.

You will be asked to wait for half an hour to see if any reactions take place. Reddening of the skin indicates that your child is allergic to that particular substance; if he is severely allergic you will see a raised white bump in the middle of the red mark. A circle guide is then placed over the bump to measure its size and, therefore, the degree of allergy the substance has triggered.

Blood tests and oxygen saturation

A RAST (radioallergosorbent) test may be used to measure allergy levels within the blood but it is not particularly specific or sensitive. The test involves taking a sample of your child's blood and sending it to a special laboratory for analysis.

A blood test may also be done to measure the concentration of certain medications in the blood. These include oral theophylline, which may be prescribed if your child's asthma is particularly bad at night.

Tests to measure oxygen levels in the blood use a non-invasive device called a pulse oximeter, which is attached to the asthma patient's finger by a special clip. It emits a beam of red light that shines through the finger and measures the color of the blood. A machine converts that color reading to a measure of the blood's oxygen content. These tests—often referred to as "sat" (for saturation) tests—are simple to do and will cause no discomfort to your child.

YOU REALLY NEED TO KNOW

◆ These tests are so much a part of the lives of the hospital staff who carry them out that they often forget that you may not understand exactly what is happening and why. If in doubt, ask.

◆ Find out details of the test procedure before the appointment and tell your child. If he knows what to expect he is less likely to worry.

◆ Remember that tests related to asthma are not carried out because your child is dangerously ill but in order to identify often avoidable triggers.

Lung, skin, and blood tests

Chapter

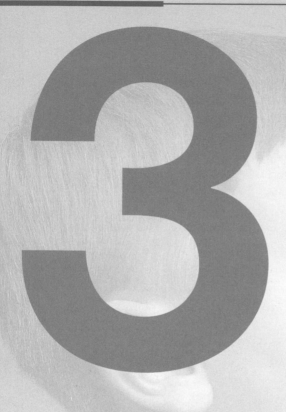

3

PREVENTION & TREATMENT

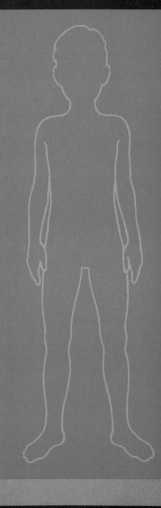

Avoiding the triggers

Thorough and frequent cleaning of the house can limit the number of dust mites.

Don't let your child be exposed to cigarette, cigar, or pipe smoke.

Don't be tempted to "improve" your house with double glazing. This will reduce the amount of air circulating, which may in turn affect your child's asthma.

The most effective way of treating your child's asthma would be to keep him away from the causes (triggers). In practice, being able to do this depends largely on what exactly the triggers are in his case, and the compromises you have to make to let him live as normal a life as possible. There are a number of simple, inexpensive steps, however, that you can take to stop your child from having "preventable" asthma attacks.

Cigarette smoke

It cannot be too highly stressed that when your child is already coping with restricted airways it is dangerous to smoke anywhere near him. It is important to make this clear to all other adults in contact with your child and, if you smoke, to get the help and advice you need to give it up. Of course all children should be discouraged from starting to smoke, especially those who have asthma.

THE IMPORTANCE OF QUITTING SMOKING

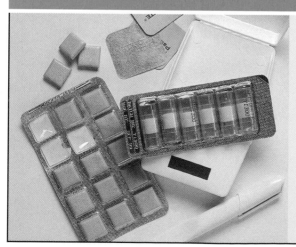

If you smoke and your child has asthma, you must quit. Breathing in your exhaled smoke makes an asthma attack far more likely. There are a number of products that can help, including nicotine patches, inhalers, and nicotine chewing gum. Discuss the best method for you with your doctor.

House dust mites

House dust mites, which form a large part of the dust in every home, are the most common asthma trigger and the one that is difficult to eradicate totally.

The mites feed off the dead skin flakes that every individual sheds almost continuously. Although these flakes are invisible to the human eye, they are very numerous. Regular cleaning means that there is less for the mites to feed on, but there are a number of other steps that can also be taken to reduce their impact.

How do I reduce dust and mites?

The first step is simply to create a few drafts. Dust mites do not flourish as readily in a well-aired home. The tendency in recent years has been to eliminate virtually all air currents, to save fuel and money. This has resulted in many homes having double-glazed windows, sealed chimneys, and wall-to-wall carpets throughout.

There are a few simple steps that you can take to increase the movement of air without increasing your heat consumption. When your carpets age, remove and do not replace them. Put down a vinyl covering or seal wooden floors so they are easy to mop. Buy cotton rugs you can wash or take outside to clean. Open windows every day to let fresh air circulate.

Without carpets in the house, you may have to wear an extra layer of clothing, but you shouldn't need to turn the heating up. You can now wash all the floors and "damp-dust" furniture (using a damp cloth rather than a duster), which is one of the best ways of removing house dust and mites. Remember to pay special attention to areas around radiator pipes and in corners where dust and mites can be concentrated.

YOU REALLY NEED TO KNOW

◆ Studies have shown that wool carpets release house dust mites into the atmosphere more readily than synthetic carpets.

◆ Soft furnishings, such as curtains, upholstery, and cushions, also harbor dust mites.

◆ Antique furniture may be stuffed with horsehair—a very common asthma trigger.

Avoiding the triggers

Avoiding the triggers

✓ Even if you buy an expensive, anti-allergy vacuum cleaner you will still need to damp-dust floors with a mop and bucket.

✓ Wash your child's bedding frequently and air it outside as often as possible.

✓ If you are treating your child for head lice, be sure to inform the pharmacist that your child is asthmatic as some lotions trigger attacks.

Beds and bedding

Children spend more time in bed than adults do. In the past, the feathers in pillows, comforters, and cushions were thought to be the cause of many asthma reactions, but experts now believe that the dust and dust mites that collect around the feathers are often the real cause.

Unless your child is also allergic to feathers, a new feather pillow with a completely sealed casing is less likely to cause problems than an old, infrequently washed synthetic pillow. However, if your child's pillows are likely to be subjected to pillowfights or other extreme wear and tear, you would be better to opt for synthetics

KEEPING THE HOUSE CLEAN

If you have an old vacuum cleaner with a worn-out dustbag, you may be putting a percentage of the dust you have just picked up back into the air. In this case, it is worth considering replacing it with a type that doesn't have a bag or has a special filter.

These cleaners, which are usually more expensive, are promoted on "anti-allergy" grounds because they remove more dust from carpets and furnishings than conventional models.

Whatever type of cleaner you buy, you will still need to wipe all surfaces and damp-dust floors with a mop and bucket. If you choose to have sealed, washable floors, which are the most practical in the early years when your child is spending a lot of time playing on the floor, you may find that you rarely use your vacuum cleaner.

because they are easier to wash. Replacing pillows every year is recommended.

Anti-allergy comforter covers and pillowcase covers seal the comforter and pillows from mites but allow air through. Whatever type of bedding you use, air it outside as much as possible. Wash all your child's bedding frequently and turn his mattress regularly.

The best kind of bed is one on legs rather than a blocked-in divan, because the dust and mites will fall from the mattress and bedding to the floor and can be vacuumed up. Bunk beds are not a good idea since dust and mites will fall from the top to the bottom bunk.

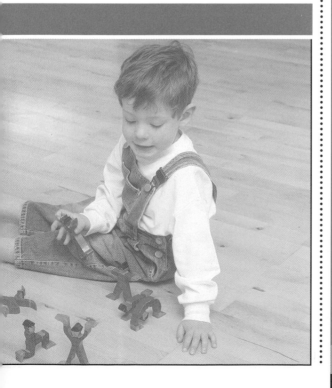

YOU REALLY NEED TO KNOW

◆ Ask the staff at hotels and holiday rentals to remove feather pillows, double-dust, and air rooms thoroughly before you arrive. Ensure the accommodation is for non-smokers.

◆ Special dust mite-excluding comforters and pillowcase covers are expensive but they are especially useful for taking on vacation and when visiting friends.

◆ Don't bother with brand-name house dust mite killers. Studies have shown damp-dusting and the other cleaning measures mentioned in this book to be more effective.

Avoiding the triggers

Avoiding the triggers

✓ Putting soft toys in the freezer for a couple of hours will help to eliminate dust mites.

✓ If you must have a dog, consider short-hair breeds, which do not shed their fur, such as poodles or schnauzers.

✓ Remember that even if you do get rid of a pet, it will take some time before all traces of it are removed from the house.

✗ Don't let pets climb on furniture or go into your child's bedroom.

Soft furnishings and toys

It is best to keep soft furnishings, draped fabrics, and dust-harboring clutter to a minimum in the bedroom, to discourage house dust mites. If your child suffers repeated bouts of asthma that you suspect are triggered by house dust mites, it is probably also worth reducing them in the rooms in which she spends most of her time, perhaps by replacing curtains with blinds and removing cushions. Fortunately you don't need to go as far as forbidding all cuddly toys. Frequent washing, preferably in hot water, is the answer and if you occasionally put the toys in plastic bags in the freezer for a couple of hours this will eradicate any mites they are harboring.

BEING AT HOME WITH PETS

Animal hair is a common asthma trigger. If you already have a much-loved pet when asthma first becomes a problem, don't rush into getting rid of the animal. You need to discuss with your doctor how seriously your child is likely to be affected by its presence. The trauma of losing the pet could also cause your child to have an asthma attack, so you need to consider the situation carefully before making a decision.

MINIMIZE THE RISKS

Remember to brush the animal outside the house every day to remove excess hair and dust (which it would otherwise shed indoors). Guinea pigs and rabbits should live in outside hutches and your child should not cuddle or handle them too much.

Indoor dampness

Damp living conditions can trigger an attack in susceptible individuals, when mold-producing spores aggravate sensitive airways. If your living area is damp, and it is impossible to eliminate the cause, open windows as much as possible to air rooms (except when the pollen count is high) and take bedding outside (or hang it out of the window) whenever the weather is dry to air it thoroughly. Keep your child's clothes and nightwear away from damp walls.

Look out for green and black spots in damp areas and wipe them away with a mild bleach solution. If possible, buy a dehumidifier to help dry out the air inside.

FINDING AN ALTERNATIVE

Fortunately it is possible to find some pets that are unlikely to trigger an asthma attack. Your child may enjoy caring for one of the less common pets, such as salamanders, lizards, and certain insects. A goldfish in a bowl or a more elaborate aquarium with a range of different fish may also appeal—surveys have shown keeping fish to be calming, and this could be beneficial to your child. Many such pets can be kept in your child's room without risk of provoking an attack, and thus may become very special to their owner. It is worth taking advice from your local vet before buying an unusual pet because some can be expensive to purchase and feed and may require expert handling to keep them in good health. Lifespans may also be short.

YOU REALLY NEED TO KNOW

◆ Try to avoid taking your child to a house where you know there will be animals; invite people to your home instead.

◆ Proteins in the urine of rodents, such as mice, hamsters, and gerbils, can provoke an asthma attack in susceptible individuals.

◆ People who are sensitive to horse dander may suffer an asthma attack after coming into contact with the clothes of a rider.

Avoiding the triggers

Avoiding the triggers

In summer, when the pollen count is high, keep the windows closed during the day.

Among the more common foods causing allergic reaction are peanuts, eggs, certain exotic fruits, dairy products, and shellfish.

Trigger foods

Food is not a common asthma trigger but asthma symptoms can occur as part of an allergic reaction to certain foods. Whole nuts should not be given in any case to preschool-age children because of the risk of their choking, but you should also remember that children with atopic conditions are more vulnerable to nut allergies. Food manufacturers now label all foods containing nuts, but if you are buying unlabeled foods or eating out, ask about the ingredients.

Artificial colorings and additives are also triggers, so try to include as many natural, unprocessed foods as possible in your child's diet. If you suspect that certain sweets or sodas are causing attacks, avoid them. This

REDUCING POLLEN IN THE YARD

If your child's asthma is triggered by pollen, there are plenty of steps you can take to make your backyard a trigger-free zone.

REPLACE THE LAWN

It is best to get rid of the lawn completely and replace it with a concrete, stone, or paved patio. Or you can use "wet-pour" surfacing, similar to that found in some children's playgrounds. This is more yielding than concrete and is available in a range of bright colors, but it is somewhat expensive. Bark is another alternative to

grass, but it gives off a dust when it breaks down, which can also act as an irritant for some children.

LOW-POLLEN FLOWERS

There is no need to eliminate flowers, but avoid those that are pollinated by wind-borne spores. All flowers that are pollinated by bees, such as sunflowers and roses, are unlikely to cause an allergic reaction and are often among the showiest flowers. If you are not sure which types to plant, your local garden center should be able to help.

will not only help you decide whether there is a problem, but also limit your child's intake of "junk" food.

Dairy products are often connected with allergies, especially eczema, but you should always ask your doctor's advice before removing them from a child's diet.

Outdoor triggers

Mold spores can be a problem outside when the weather is damp, especially in autumn when vegetation is dying off. Teach your child to keep away from the compost pile if you have one. Put up fences rather than hedges to mark boundaries if you can because mold spores collect in hedges.

Ways of avoiding pollen

Pollen is very difficult to avoid during the summer months. The worst time is early summer when so many plants are in flower. Rain literally washes pollen away, so the pollen count is highest during a dry spell and you may have to be extra vigilant at this time. Get into the habit of finding out about the daily pollen count, then plan your child's activities accordingly.

Encourage him to play outside only when the pollen count is lower, which is early in the morning or just before bed. Resist the temptation to bring cut flowers inside the house. Open windows and doors to air the house early in the morning and then keep them closed for the rest of the day. Do not hang clothes outside to dry or bedding to air when the pollen count is high.

If your child reacts badly to pollen, ask his school if he can stay inside at times when there is a high pollen count and when the grass has just been cut. Remind him never to roll in grass, even when he sees his friends doing it.

YOU REALLY NEED TO KNOW

◆ Peanut butter and crude peanut oil must be eliminated from the diets of children who are allergic to nuts. Purified peanut oil, however, is safe.

◆ If your child is allergic to peanuts or nuts, ask a dietician for advice on how to avoid them totally. They are present in a surprising number of processed foods.

◆ When the pollen count is high, consider spending a family day at the beach rather than in the country.

Avoiding the triggers

Medication—inhalers

SELF-HELP

✓ Make sure your child carries his inhaler with him at all times.

✓ If you understand how an inhaler is supposed to work, you will know if your child is using it correctly.

✓ Novelty plastic covers depicting favorite cartoon characters can make inhalers more child-friendly.

Inhalers—often known as puffers—are the most common means of taking asthma medication. They consist of a small aerosol canister of the prescribed drug inside a plastic sleeve with a mouthpiece and a removable cap to keep the mouthpiece clean and free from dust. They can be used alone or with a holding chamber (see p. 53).

How to use a metered-dose inhaler

First shake the inhaler, then hold it with the canister pointing upward like a periscope and the mouthpiece at the bottom. Remove the cap and, after breathing out, make an airtight seal with your mouth around the mouthpiece. As you breathe in, press the canister down into the covering so that a measured dose of the drug is released through the mouthpiece. Continue to breathe in until you have taken a full breath.

The medication comes out in a fine mist through a tiny hole. It is important to coordinate the release of the mist with breathing in, so that all of the drug is taken into the lungs. Finally, hold your breath for as long as possible.

Choosing the best method

It is essential that children use a device that is suited to their age since this ensures that the correct amount of the drug reaches their lungs and makes it more likely that they will use the medication correctly. Dry-powder devices can be used from around five years upward and may be easier to use at school. These are available in the form of round disks or spinhalers. Both work in a similar fashion. Either a push of a lever on the disk or a twist of the spinhaler loads a measured dose of powder medication that is inhaled in a deep breath, followed by holding in the breath for as long as possible.

Make medication a part of daily life

If your child is very young, it is a good idea to keep his inhalers and holding chamber, or spacer, where he can see them and become familiar with them, but cannot play with them. The equipment should soon become an accepted part of daily life, since hiding them away and producing them only when it is time to use them may well act as a signal for a confrontation.

USING AN INHALER

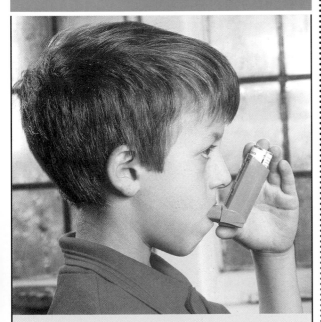

By about the age of ten, your child will probably be coordinated enough to use an inhaler for a metered dose. Some inhalers may be used with a holding chamber or spacer (see p. 53).

(see p. 53)

YOU REALLY NEED TO KNOW

◆ The inhaler should be shaken before each use so that the propellant mixes with the drug. If the propellant sinks to the bottom, your child will receive more propellant than medication.

◆ Remove the tube of medication from time to time and wash the plastic casing. This prevents a build-up of medication and ensures the fine mist comes through efficiently.

◆ Always have a spare inhaler so that your child never runs out of medication.

Medication—inhalers

Medication—for intervention

Bronchodilators are drugs that relieve your child's symptoms. They are the front-line medication for asthma symptoms. All sufferers of asthma should have an inhaler available at all times. Side-effects are rare, but if your child does experience any, you should consult your doctor

METHODS TO RELIEVE ASTHMA ATTACKS	
TYPE	**GENERIC NAME**
BRONCHODILATORS, ALSO CALLED BETA-ADRENERGIC AGONISTS (INHALERS, PILLS, OR NEBULIZERS)	albuterol terbutaline metaproterenol
METHYL-XANTHINES (PILLS, LIQUID, OR CAPSULES)	theophylline aminophylline
INJECTIONS	epinephrine ipratropium

These medications are best given via inhaler or can be taken via a nebulizer, particularly in more severe episodes.

EFFECTS/USES	POSSIBLE SIDE-EFFECTS
First choice of treatment in most cases. Open up constricted airways to relieve wheezing and asthma symptoms. Available in inhaler, liquid, and nebulizer form.	• Hyperactivity • Headaches • Hand tremor • Fast heart rate
Effective bronchodilators but less effective than beta-agonists. Side-effects affect 10–15 percent of children. Blood tests of levels are necessary.	• Nausea • Vomiting • Stomach pain • Headaches • Hyperactivity • Distractability
These days primarily used for infants.	• Racing heart

For babies and young children who do not yet have the coordination to use an inhaler, liquid is available.

YOU REALLY NEED TO KNOW

◆ Bronchodilators are used for relief at the onset of symptoms. If you think an attack is predictable, for example, if exercise is a trigger, your child should use her inhaler fifteen minutes before the exercise session starts.

◆ Brochodilators work within fifteen minutes and the effects last for about four hours. If you see no improvement or your child's condition worsens, it is a sign of a moderately severe asthma attack. Consult your doctor.

◆ Bronchodilators are misused the most often. Have regular good practice updates with your child and keep in touch with your asthma clinic.

Medication—for intervention

Medication—for maintenance

A holding chamber can be used with an inhaler if your child finds it difficult to use.

Don't allow your child and his friends to play with his inhalers.

Don't keep inhalers hidden from view. The more familiar your child is with this important equipment the more likely he is to accept it.

Drugs designed to prevent asthma attacks are an important part of your child's medication. Many parents may feel concerned about their child taking regular doses of drugs, even when he shows no sign of illness. But for the child with asthma, preventive medication can be the most effective and least stressful and damaging course of action.

Taking regular doses from a maintenance inhaler doesn't mean that your child will lose his chance of growing out of asthma, nor does it mean that he will become addicted, needing even higher doses. Fewer asthma attacks mean less strain on his respiratory system and less disruption of day-to-day activities. Your doctor will only prescribe the absolute minimum dose needed to keep your child healthy and you can discuss decreasing the dose as and when your child's symptoms lessen.

How to use a maintenance inhaler

Your doctor will give you instructions about when your child should use this inhaler. It is common for it to be given just before meals or before your child brushes his teeth, to make timing easier to remember. If your child is young, you can use a spacer, just as you can with a reliever inhaler.

You may find that because this medication has to be taken regularly every day even when your child is symptom-free, you meet with some resistance. When a child has asthma symptoms he usually cooperates because he knows that using his inhaler will make him feel better. When he hasn't any symptoms he may not want to take his medicine. You can help by explaining that using this particular inhaler will keep him feeling well because it reduces inflammation in his lungs.

HOW A SPACER HELPS

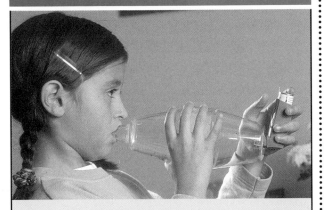

A holding chamber is a long, rounded plastic device that comes in two halves. There is a hole in one end of one part, where the inhaler fits in, and a mouthpiece in front of a valve at the other. The two parts fit together.

Children under ten can find it difficult to press an inhaler and breathe in at the same time. A holding chamber helps a child to obtain the medication needed.

HOW DOES A HOLDING CHAMBER WORK?

When a puff of medication is released from the inhaler into the chamber this gives your child time to breathe calmly and take the dose in. You will hear the valve click as this happens so you know the medication is being received. Your child should repeat five deep, slow breaths with each puff of medication.

With babies or children under the age of two or three years, it is easier to use a soft face mask with a smaller chamber—you hold the chamber at 45 degrees, keeping the mask in place for 30 seconds (see p. 60).

(see p. 60)

3

YOU REALLY NEED TO KNOW

◆ Maintenance inhalers are designed to prevent attacks from happening and to reduce the frequency of attacks.

◆ Organize medication for the same times each day. It may be useful to introduce a "reward" scheme if your child is reluctant to take his medication.

◆ When you are going on vacation ensure you have enough inhalers to last your entire stay.

Medication—for maintenance

There are a number of drugs that prevent asthma attacks. The type your doctor prescribes will depend on the severity of your child's asthma.

DRUGS TO PREVENT ASTHMA ATTACKS	
TYPE	**GENERIC NAME**
INHALED ANTI-INFLAMMATORIES	cromolyn sodium nedocromil
INHALED CORTICOSTEROIDS (USUALLY JUST CALLED STEROIDS)	beclomethasone dipropionat flunisolide
ORAL STEROIDS (see p. 56)	hydrocortisone prednisone methyl prednisolone dexamethasone

EFFECTS/USES	POSSIBLE SIDE-EFFECTS
• To prevent irritation of the airways. • To inhibit the production of mucus, which would clog the airways. • Needs to be taken two to four times a day.	• Coughing
• For more serious asthma or at a time when triggers are prevalent. • Needs to be taken twice a day.	• Hoarseness • Oral thrush
• Short course rescue therapy given as liquid or pills.	

YOU REALLY NEED TO KNOW

◆ Steroid drugs are inhaled in small amounts through an inhaler, and are very effective. The dose given is unlikely to cause any long-term side-effects. After use, it is important to rinse the mouth and spit out to reduce the risk further.

◆ If your child is using her preventer properly she will need to use her reliever a lot less and not at all on most days.

◆ Asthma that is not properly controlled is far more likely to inhibit a child's growth than taking the correct doses of medication.

Other medication

Inhalers are the most effective way of giving most asthma medication, but it may also be given in liquid or pill form. A very young child who finds it difficult to use an inhaler, even with a spacer, may temporarily be prescribed a medication in liquid form.

As well as the inhaled steroids, there are some medications that are taken as pills or liquid to provide additional beneficial effects. The group, called theophyllines, may be prescribed to control difficult symptoms, for example, at night. There are some side-effects that may occur, including nausea, vomiting, and interaction with other medication. It is important that you talk to your doctor about this so you know what to expect and what you might have to do if they occur.

Oral steroids

Sometimes your child may need to take oral steroids to help get her asthma back under control, for example, when she has a bad cold or other asthma triggers to deal with. This should not happen often, providing you stick to your asthma management plan. If it does happen more often than you expect, you should not consider it a failure on your part or as something that could cause problems for your child's long-term health.

Your doctor will only prescribe oral steroids if there is a danger of the asthma becoming out of control without them. Short courses are very safe. Usually, when a child takes oral steroids her condition improves dramatically in a short period of time.

The oral steroids prescribed for children are hydrocortisone, prednisone, methyl prednisolone, and dexamethasone. For young children these are usually given as liquid. Have a drink ready because your child will probably want to wash away the taste of the medication. Older children may prefer to swallow pills.

Treating a severe attack

In the rare event that your child needs to stay in the hospital, she will almost certainly be given steroids. If she has been admitted with a severe attack the medication may be given intravenously through a small plastic tube inserted into her arm. This may look dramatic, but giving medication intravenously is simply an effective method of getting the drug to act quickly.

If your child receives intravenous medication she will probably need to complete a course of oral steroids at home. In rare and very severe cases, oral steroids are taken on a long-term basis, preferably on alternate days.

IMMUNOTHERAPY

Immunotherapy consists of an injection, or course of injections, of a diluted allergen (allergy-causing) solution. The solution acts like a vaccine to neutralize an allergy and is usually considered when an individual suffers badly from one single allergy. The treatment is usually carried out at a specialist's allergy clinic because of the possible side-effect of an induced asthma attack.

If your child suffers from one of the atopic conditions often associated with asthma and there is a strong probability that her asthma is triggered by a single allergy, it may be worth talking to your doctor about the possibility of immunotherapy. It is seldom considered useful for children, however, as they often grow out of asthma.

YOU REALLY NEED TO KNOW

◆ Short courses of oral steroids will not affect your child's growth and development. Occasional courses of steroid pills or liquid have a very low risk of side-effects.

◆ Studies have shown that uncontrolled asthma contributes more to growth retardation than using steroid-based medication.

◆ Very few asthmatic children need long courses of oral steroids, but if your child does, her growth and development will be closely monitored and the dose reduced as quickly as possible.

Other medication

Nebulizers

SELF-HELP

✓ Keep nebulizer face masks and tubes clean and replace them every few months.

✓ Sit with your child while he uses the nebulizer and make sure he inhales the full dose.

A nebulizer runs off a small compressor powered by electricity and is used either in a hospital or at home to treat more severe attacks. Liquid medication is poured into the reservoir of the nebulizer, and either air or oxygen is blown through the liquid to produce a fine mist. Your child then inhales this mist through a face mask or, preferably, a mouthpiece.

It can be very useful, but there are disadvantages: for example, the noise the machine makes in use, the time taken to administer the medication, and its weight and size which make it less portable than other devices.

THE BEST WAY OF USING A NEBULIZER

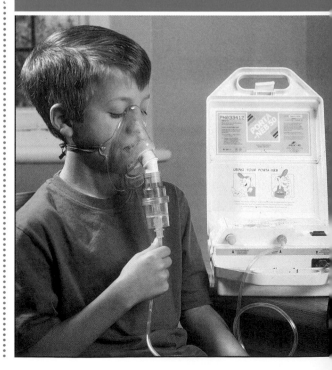

Keeping a nebulizer at home

If your child is very young and has already had several severe asthma attacks, or if there is more than one asthmatic in your family, it is worth considering keeping a nebulizer at home. Your doctor will be able to advise you whether this is necessary in your case.

You will need to keep the face mask and tube clean and dust-free and replace them every few months. Most of the companies that supply nebulizers provide stickers of favorite cartoon characters to make the machine more appealing to a child.

When your child has to use a nebulizer, you can help by making the experience as comfortable as possible. You will be more prepared if you know what to expect. It is important that your child sits still and inhales all of the dose. He may be able to sit on your lap or next to you so you can cuddle him. You will have the noise of the machine and the sound of the medication vaporizing inside the mask to contend with. This will make it difficult to read aloud to your child or carry on a conversation. It could be useful to have some brightly illustrated picture books to look through during the time it takes, usually about ten minutes.

3

YOU REALLY NEED TO KNOW

◆ Some hospitals loan nebulizers to asthmatic patients for home use—ask at yours if this is possible.

◆ When not in use the nebulizer should be stored in its own carrying case.

◆ If you are planning to take a nebulizer abroad, check whether you will need to take an adaptor for the plug.

Nebulizers

Using medication

The type of medication your child needs and the delivery device to use depends on his age, how serious his condition is, and how well he responds to treatment.

Babies

It is not uncommon for parents to feel downhearted if their baby succumbs to an attack. Instead of imagining he will be ill for the rest of his life, reassure yourself that even babies with very severe asthma can outgrow the condition by the time they start school. Just growing physically larger is what helps many children.

Nevertheless, it is vital that your baby receives the necessary medication at the correct moment. Mild asthma may require a bronchodilator, such as albuterol or terbutaline. Serious asthma that is affected by recurrent colds and infections may need both a bronchodilator and a steroid medication.

WHEN A BABY HAS ASTHMA

A baby with severe asthma will need more than one medication to control his condition. The best way to deliver these is via a holding chamber and face mask. If this is difficult, a nebulizer can be used. Short courses of liquid steroids may be another solution.

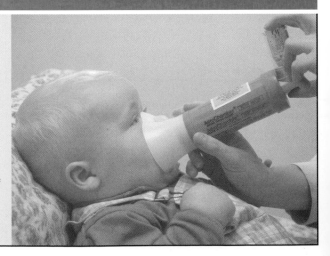

Preschoolers

Preschool children are old enough to put up resistance but not mature enough to understand why they need medication. Your child will use a holding chamber with an inhaler at this stage, preferably with a mouthpiece rather than a mask since this is more effective. Turning your child's medication time into a "fun" session may help you to avoid tantrums. This obviously works better when neither you nor your child is overtired or upset.

Schoolchildren

This may be the first time you have delegated your child's care and are not supervising his medication at all times. He will be more active and new routines at school may put him under stress. This is the time to make doubly sure you keep to good asthma habits at home and encourage your child to accept his inhaler routine as an ordinary part of daily life. A regular appointment at the doctor's office is still necessary to monitor and adjust the dosage.

Older children

As children approach their teens they tend to pay less attention to what their parents say; this includes advice on medication. As your child is now more likely to be involved in serious sports, years of good practice should make him recognize the need to carry his inhaler in his kit. He is also increasingly likely to stay away from home overnight so you should tell other parents about his inhalers in the same way that you would explain special dietary requirements. Though children hate to be seen to be different, this should never be accepted as an excuse for not keeping up with the inhaler routine.

3

**YOU REALLY
NEED TO KNOW**

◆ If your child takes longer than normal to respond to his inhaler or you notice he is starting to use it up faster, his condition needs to be reassessed.

◆ Most parents worry about the side-effects of asthma medication, but the side-effect of a serious, untreated asthma attack is potentially far worse. With proper guidance, medication will enhance your child's life.

◆ Most pediatricians are concerned about getting asthma care right. Find a doctor your child likes and whom you respect.

Using medication

Chapter

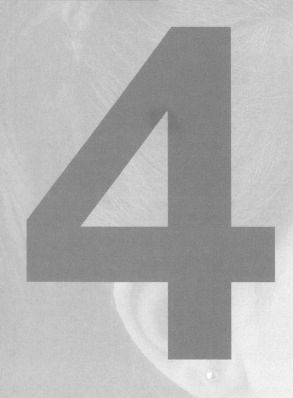

4

DAY-TO-DAY CARE

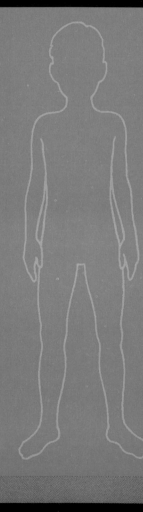

What are the danger signs?

SELF-HELP

✓ Stay close to your child during an attack to help calm her.

✗ It is natural for you to feel anxious, but try to conceal this from your child to avoid upsetting her further.

No matter how well you seem to have your child's asthma under control, there is always the risk of an acute attack. You need to be aware of the warning signs so that you can take prompt action.

A key sign is that her normal medication doesn't seem to be working as well as usual. Other signs that her asthma may be getting out of control include having to take her reliever medication more frequently, wheezing constantly, being short of breath and unable to complete her sentences, coughing persistently, breathing at an increased rate, feeling tired, and looking very pale. A severe head cold or other viral infection of the upper respiratory tract are common triggers.

THE SIGNS OF AN IMMINENT ATTACK

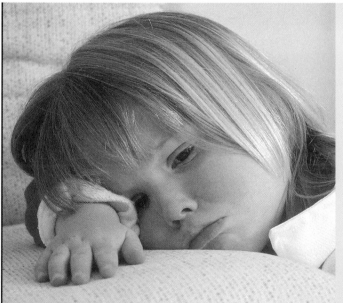

You may find that your child becomes tired and listless. She may have a cold. She may look much paler than usual. Her normal medication may not be working as well and more inhaler may be needed. She may breathe faster, be short of breath, wheeze, and cough.

How can I help my child?

If your child is wheezing, encourage her to breathe deeply and slowly, although not so deeply that it will bring on a fit of coughing. Try to remain calm and be as reassuring as possible. Remember any fear you feel is easily transmitted to your child and this is likely to make the wheezing even worse.

Acute attacks frequently happen at night. Your child will find it easier to breathe if she is sitting up, with you close by to hold her hand or put your arm around her. This will help to calm her while she tries to get her breathing under control.

What else can I do?

You should try to prevent her from becoming dehydrated. Encourage her to sip small amounts at frequent intervals. Plain water is best, although juice is popular with some children at these times. Provide a straw if that makes it easier for her to drink. She might like to suck a piece of ice.

Don't worry if she doesn't feel like eating—you can offer food once the attack has passed. If she has swallowed a lot of mucus or is coughing, she may vomit, which may make her feel better.

Even if the symptoms improve, it is a good idea to contact your doctor. Once the attack is over it can help to look back on why and how it happened. You may be surprised at how many signs there were during the days leading up to the attack. If it followed on from an accumulation of factors, such as watching sports in cold conditions, a succession of late nights that led to haphazard taking of preventive medication, you may be able to act to prevent a similar pattern from recurring.

4

YOU REALLY NEED TO KNOW

The symptoms which herald an acute asthma attack and demand immediate action promptly are:

◆ Wheezing.

◆ Shortness of breath.

◆ Persistent coughing.

◆ Increased breathing rate.

◆ Inability to speak or complete a sentence.

What are the danger signs?

When is it an emergency?

✓ Make sure you know the danger signs so you can call for help as soon as it is needed.

✓ Let the emergency medical services (EMS) know what you have noticed about your child's condition.

✗ Don't panic. No matter how difficult it is, try to appear calm to avoid alarming your child further.

Parents and care givers of a child with asthma should be aware that it is not uncommon for an acute attack to develop into a medical emergency. Recent research showed that one in five children who had had asthma diagnosed by their doctor had to be hospitalized at some point. A serious deterioration in your child's condition is a frightening experience for you and your child and it is essential that you recognize when it is time to call for help.

What should I look out for?

Long before an emergency situation develops, it is vital that you know what the signs of deterioration are and how to react to them. If your child's symptoms are not improving and she is exhausted by the very effort of breathing, she should be seen by a doctor as soon as possible.

Her breathing will become very rapid. As it becomes increasingly labored, the whole of her upper body will appear to be involved in the struggle. The space between her ribs, the bottom of the ribcage, and the area above her collarbone will all appear to be sucked in with every breath she takes.

The wheezing may have become less obvious but this may be more a sign of fatigue than improvement in her condition. Though it is less noisy, it can be an indication that her breathing is becoming more shallow and this means she is taking less oxygen into her bloodstream. She may become unable to speak sentences and may also have chest pains.

How long will she stay in the hospital?

Children usually recover very quickly from attacks such as these once the asthma has been controlled by emergency action. Sufferers rarely spend more than one or two nights in the hospital. While your child is there the doctors may do some tests, such as a chest X ray, to eliminate any other causes for the breathing difficulty.

IN AN EMERGENCY

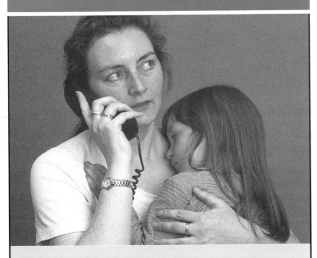

◆ PHONE FOR AN AMBULANCE immediately if you notice that your child's lips, tongue, or fingernails show any bluish tinge.

◆ TELL THE EMERGENCY SERVICE about your child's condition: How she is breathing, her skin color, etc., so that they arrive fully equipped to deal with the crisis.

◆ STAY WITH YOUR CHILD. All her body systems are deprived of oxygen and are starting to slow down. Her condition is now life-threatening.

◆ EMERGENCY ACTION: Your child will immediately be given oxygen. Once she reaches the hospital, anti-asthma drugs may be given intravenously. She may also be put on a drip to replace any fluid lost through dehydration.

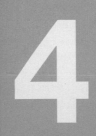

YOU REALLY NEED TO KNOW

These are the signs that your child's condition is now very serious and needs immediate medical attention:

◆ Her peak flow is one third of normal.

◆ She is unable to speak.

◆ She has chest pains.

◆ Her breathing has become shallow.

◆ Her lips, tongue, or fingernails are turning blue.

◆ Her level of awareness drops, or she loses consciousness.

When is it an emergency?

Help him to help himself

Despite the fact that asthma is becoming increasingly common, some children with the condition do feel isolated and different from their friends. It is important that you do everything you can to dispel these feelings and help your child to live as normal a life as possible.

Apart from the times when your child feels really unwell, there is no reason why he shouldn't do all the things other children do. If your child finds himself constantly excluded from activities that he sees others enjoying, he will feel miserable and depressed, so it is

ENCOURAGE YOUR CHILD'S INDEPENDENCE

Feeling very protective toward your child is understandable, particularly after several acute attacks. It is, however, important to see him as an indivdual. Resist any temptation to fuss. Making your child feel like an invalid could seriously affect his self-esteem and delay his emotional and social development.

There is also the danger that if you are overanxious he may take a cue from you and become constantly fearful. Or he may use the asthma as an excuse to get out of doing things he could easily do but doesn't want to.

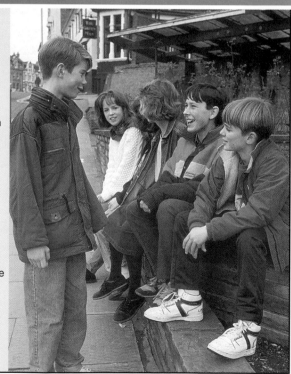

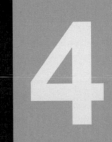

4

essential that he be allowed to play and take part in other physical activities just like everyone else.

Let him take responsibility

A child with asthma needs to take responsibility for his own health from an early age since you will not always be with him to detect the signs of an imminent attack.

He must be taught to recognize when his asthma is getting out of control and be fully knowledgeable about his medication. He will soon learn to predict when an attack of wheezing is about to happen and when he needs to use his inhaler. He also needs to be sure in his own mind of the things that are likely to trigger an attack so that he can avoid them as far as possible or take extra medication should avoidance be impossible.

Being kept fully informed and given responsibility for the management of his own condition from an early age will help him to cope even if he has a severe attack. Discuss any changes in his care plan with him and always encourage him to ask questions.

He should become involved in the discussions you have with the doctor about his asthma as soon as you feel he is old enough to understand what is being said. Even a very young child can quickly become an expert on his own condition.

Problems with an older child

You may find that as your child gets older and becomes more image conscious he starts to refuse to take his medication to school and is reluctant to use an inhaler in front of friends in case they see it as a sign of weakness. Even if he does take the medication with him, he may decide not to take it. You may need a new strategy.

Help him to help himself

DOs AND DON'Ts

✓ Join a support group to meet other people in your situation.

✗ Don't let your child stop taking preventer medication without medical advice, even if he hasn't had an asthma attack for a long time.

Will changing his regime help?

If your child begins to get really careless about taking medication at school, ask your doctor about changing the regime. Some asthma medications are given four times a day, but a double dose twice a day may be possible.

If he has not had an attack for a long time it may be appropriate to stop taking medicine and to rely on inhalers to treat symptoms. If so, stress how important it is that he takes his medication when needed because this is the only way his asthma can be properly managed.

It is worrisome to have a child who suddenly becomes blasé about his condition but this can and does happen, particularly as the child approaches his teens. At this stage, peer pressure, a need to feel the same as others, and a desire to be independent all become issues. Try to be as supportive and understanding as you can.

Where can I get help?

If your child does find it hard to come to terms with his condition, you may find it helpful to contact a support group through which both you and he can form relationships with other families who are in a similar position. As your child gets older he might enjoy going to a specialized summer camp where he can meet children with the same problems and find out how they cope.

What about the future?

With careful monitoring and regular medication, asthma can now be very successfully managed. In most cases there is no reason why it should restrict your child's life or affect his long-term health in any major way. If your child is one of the lucky ones, he may even outgrow the condition by the time he reaches puberty.

WHY IS EXERCISE IMPORTANT?

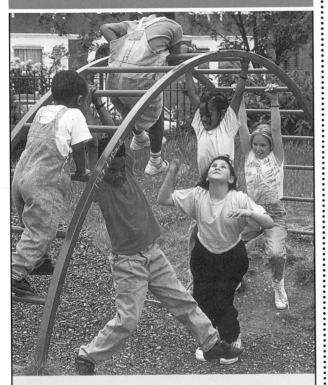

Exercise is vital to your child's wellbeing. It promotes the growth of healthy bones and helps to maintain a strong heart and lungs. Even a child whose asthma is exercise-induced should be allowed to take part in sports and other physical activities, as long as he always has an inhaler with him and uses it promptly to reverse an attack. Both you and your child should be encouraged by the long list of men and women who have been very successful in athletics and other sports, such as soccer and swimming, despite their asthma.

**YOU REALLY
NEED TO KNOW**

◆ Teach your child to recognize his own particular warning signs or, if this is difficult, to use his peak flow meter to monitor his condition.

◆ Encourage your child to write down the time he uses his inhaler. If he needs to use his inhaler more often than every four hours, the asthma attack is moderately severe and he should see his doctor.

◆ Suggest activities like swimming and yoga because they build up strength in the lungs and help with breathing.

Help him to help himself

Whom should I tell?

SELF-HELP

Keep the school fully informed about your child's condition.

Make sure your child knows that she can use her inhaler up to every four hours.

Give the school a peak flow meter like the one you use at home, with the normal and danger levels clearly marked.

When your child starts school you will probably feel nervous at the thought of not being around all the time to make sure she takes her medication or to detect the signs of an imminent attack. Because asthma is so common, most teachers will be familiar to some extent with the condition. However, since it varies so much in severity from child to child, you shouldn't rely on your child's teacher to have the knowledge to deal with her individual needs.

Before your child starts at any new school you should arrange a meeting with her class teacher. He or she should also arrange for you to meet any other members of the staff who will spend time with your child and who will need to know about her asthma. This will include non-teaching staff who will be responsible for your child during lunch breaks and playtimes and perhaps on trips away from school.

What should I tell the school?

You should provide the school with clear, written details of your child's medication and the things that are likely to trigger an attack. Schools can be full of potential triggers, such as chalk dust, and chemicals used during science lessons. You need to impress upon the school staff that your child must use her inhaler immediately if there is any sign of wheezing or shortness of breath. You should also ensure that the school has up-to-date written details of your telephone number and the name and number of your child's doctor.

Where will the medication be kept?

Schools vary in their policies about where inhalers and other medications are kept. Your child needs to know that she can have access to her inhaler whenever she needs it and who she should approach to get it.

Problems can arise at break time, particularly on very cold days. Your child may panic if she is outside and her inhaler is locked away inside the school building. This is why auxiliary staff looking after children during non-teaching time need to realize how important it is for asthma sufferers to be given medication when they need it, and what they should do in an emergency.

COPING WITH ASTHMA AT SCHOOL

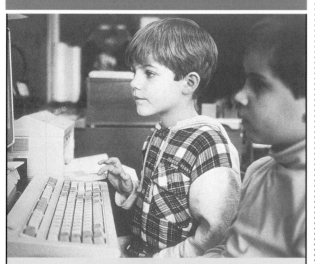

Your child's school will have a clear policy on where medication is kept, how its use is recorded, and who is allowed to administer it. A child who understands all these ground rules will be able to concentrate on schoolwork, secure in the knowledge that help will be given should an asthma attack seem imminent.

YOU REALLY NEED TO KNOW

Keep your child at home if:

◆ The wheezing continues after she has taken her medication.

◆ There is any sign of possible infection, such as a sore throat or swollen glands.

◆ She seems hot and feverish.

◆ She seems unusually tired.

Whom should I tell?

Whom should I tell?

DOs AND DON'Ts

Find out what is causing any anxiety because it might trigger asthma attacks.

Don't let your child get away with bad behavior because of her asthma.

How can the teachers help?

Teachers are encouraged to work in partnership with parents on all aspects of school life, including health issues. It will also help your child's academic progress if you can develop a close relationship with her teachers. If she does have to take time off from school you will then be able to talk to them about what work can be completed at home. You can obtain information packs designed specifically for teachers to help them and their other pupils understand asthma and its implications.

What if the teacher is unhelpful?

Occasionally an asthmatic child may come up against an unsympathetic teacher, who can seriously dent her confidence. If she suddenly becomes very anxious when

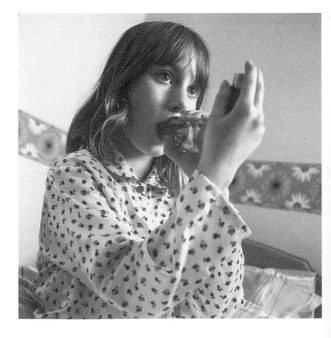

An older child will gradually gain more independence, including staying overnight with friends. Ask her friends' parents not to treat her differently, but make sure they know the signs that an attack is imminent.

it's time for school, which in itself can bring on an asthma attack, you need to investigate possible causes and discuss the matter with the school principal. While you need to feel confident that your child is well cared for, you also have to make it clear to the school that you are not asking for special treatment and that she should not be routinely excluded from any activity. Nor should she be allowed to use her asthma as an excuse for bad behavior.

Staying away from home

As your child gets older she will want to have more independence and start doing things on her own, such as visiting friends' homes and staying overnight. This may cause you some anxiety, but you would feel even more concerned if she were not being invited to parties and sleepovers because her friends' parents felt unable to cope should she have an acute asthma attack.

Visits to other people's homes will probably require some preplanning, particularly if it means your child will come up against common triggers, such as pets or feather bedding. She may be able to overcome the pet problem by taking extra medication, although if the presence of a cat or dog makes her feel really ill she probably won't enjoy the social occasion. If she is invited to sleep at a friend's house, ask the parents if she can bring her own pillow and sleeping bag.

What about the future?

An asthmatic child must be allowed to lead as full a life as any other child. If you have ensured that your child and everyone else responsible for her care are fully informed about her condition and that her medication is readily available, she can face the world with confidence.

YOU REALLY NEED TO KNOW

◆ Just because your child has asthma, it doesn't mean she must live an overprotected life.

◆ Provided she and everyone else responsible for her care are fully informed about her condition and know what to do in an emergency, she can be treated the same as any other child.

◆ Independence is as important for an asthmatic child as it is for any other, so you need to play your part in helping her to achieve it.

Whom should I tell?

Understanding the jargon

Many of the terms you will meet when finding out more about your child's asthma may be unfamiliar to you. This page gives some definitions, and on page 78 you will find addresses of useful contact groups.

ALLERGENS—substances that cause an allergic reaction in susceptible individuals. They can be absorbed through breathing, contact with the skin, or by eating certain foods.

ACUTE ASTHMA—a condition that occurs when the normal medication fails to work and an actual attack occurs. Wheezing becomes very obvious and your child has difficulty breathing out.

BRONCHODILATOR—a drug treatment that helps ease constriction in the airways during an attack of asthma.

BRONCHODILATOR INHALERS—a drug treatment that alleviates symptoms when an asthma attack has started.

CHRONIC ASTHMA—a condition where the inflammation in the lungs means that there is always likely to be some wheezing and coughing and the possibility of an acute attack.

CYANOSIS—a dangerous condition in which a reduction of oxygen in the blood leads to blueness around the lips, tongue, and fingernails.

DECONGESTANTS—drugs used to relieve mucus or congestion in the nose.

EXERCISE-INDUCED ASTHMA—an attack brought on by strenuous physical activity.

EXTRINSIC ASTHMA—a condition in which something like pollen, house dust and mites, or animal fur is the trigger for an attack. It can be an inherited condition, particularly if one or both parents suffer allergies.

HOLDING CHAMBER—a round or tube-shaped device attached to the end of an inhaler in which medication in mist form collects before it is breathed in.

INTRINSIC ASTHMA—a condition that can be caused by a viral infection, cold air, or exercise.

MAINTENANCE INHALER—a drug treatment that reduces inflammation in the airways and must be taken on a regular basis whether or not your child is having any symptoms.

MUCOSA—the lining of the airways that contains mucus-producing glands.

NEBULIZER—equipment that enables medication to be given in a mist form. The child breathes it in by using a mouthpiece or a face mask.

PEAK FLOW METER—a device for measuring how well your child's lungs are working.

PULMONARY FUNCTION TESTS—tests carried out by asking the patient to blow into a machine called a spirometer to see how well he can breathe out.

TRIGGER—anything that sets off an asthma attack.

WHEEZE—a high pitched, whistling noise.

Useful addresses

CANADIAN PEDIATRIC SOCIETY
Ms Nicole Menzies – Chief
Administrative Officer
100 - 2204 Walkley Road
Ottawa, ON
KIG 4G8
Telephone: (613) 526-9397
Fax (613) 526-3332
E-mail: nicolem@cps.ca
Web Site: www.cps.ca

**CHILDREN'S HOSPITAL OF
EASTERN ONTARIO**
401 Smyth Road
Ottawa, ON
K1H 8L1
Telephone: (613) 737-7600
CHEO Health Information Line
(613) 738-4888

**THE LUNG ASSOCIATION,
NATIONAL OFFICE**
1900 City Park Drive, Suite 508
Gloucester, ON
K1J 1A3
Telephone (613) 747-6776
Fax: (613) 747-7430
Canadian Lung Association:
http://www.lung.ca/asthma/

ASTHMA CENTRE
The Toronto Hospital
Western Division
399 Bathurst Street
4 ECW
Toronto, ON
M5T 2S8
E-mail: care@asthmacentre.com

USEFUL WEBSITES
Health Canada Online:
http://www.hc-sc.gc.ca/

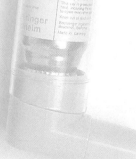

Index

Index

Acknowledgments
Photographs: Collections: Lesley Howling: 27; A. Sieveking: 64;
B. Shuel: 68; Corbis: 23, 29, 44-45; Guglielmo Galvin: 35, 49, 53, 58; Sally & Richard
Greenhill: 20; Science Photo Library: 8-9, 15, 24, 30-31, 33, 36, 57, 62-63, 74; Andrew
Sydenham: 40; Tony Stone Images: 73; Tim Woodcock Library: 71.
All other photographs by George Taylor. Special thanks to Sue Jenkins, Matthew Coomb,
Lydia Coomb, Joe Hurst, and Lily Hurst for modeling for the photographs.
Illustration: Coral Mula: 10.